LIVING TWICE AS LONG

BY

BOBBY F. BROOKS

Prologue

If you're still young, when I say young, I mean between 45 and 55. You should be planning on living past 100 years of age. Why, because in 50 years from right now it should be commonplace for most humans in this country to live past 100 years of age. But, you've got to start right now to make it happen. Read this book to get started on your road to longevity.

Contents

Live twice as long as your ancestors.

Back in the 1900s, life expectancy was only 50 years. Of course, some people lived much longer than that. But then again many did make it to 50. Obviously, something changed between then and now. What was it?

As you can guess, there were many reasons life expectancy was so short. The main reasons were, lifestyle and diet.

Researchers from all around the world have been searching for the fountain of youth PILL forever. With today's modern medicine they have come closer than ever before of finding a formula to slow down the aging process. More about that later.

Your cardiovascular system

First, let's go over some cold hard facts. Your cardiovascular system is the most common part of your body to be affected by old age. As you get older, the blood vessels and arteries that pump blood to your heart began to stiffen, this causes your heart to work much harder to pump the blood through your cardiovascular system and as these changes take place your body is at greater risk of problems like high blood pressure typically called hypertension. As you get older, you have a much higher risk of heart disease. Later will go into what you can do to lower your risk of heart disease.

BONES, JOINTS, AND MUSCLES

The next things you notice is that your bones, joints, and muscles tend to stiffen. Did you know that with age your bones decrease in size and density? Weak bones tend to fracture more easily. And then you begin to lose flexibility and muscle strength. Don't worry will talking about what you can do to prolong all of that later.

YOUR LARGE INTESTINES

Did you know that as you get older, you tend to become constipated? It's true in most cases. That's because as you get older, there are structural changes in your large intestines that causes constipation. Later I'm going to tell you how to prevent constipation.

Do you feel the need to urinate more often? As you get older, it's a commonplace, and that's because your bladder may become less elastic with age. There's a strategy to help you with this problem, and I'll address that later on.

YOUR BRAINS AND MEMORY

As we age so do our brains. Like with everything else in our body our brains begin to change with age. Along with that change comes the possibility of memory loss. You may start to forget small things like someone's name or where you left your car keys. You'll want to learn how to keep a healthy brain.

YOUR EYES AND EARS

By middle age, you are already starting to have problems with your eyes. , Generally, the first thing that happens is you began to have problems seeing up close like trying to remove the splinter from your finger or threading the needle. Then you notice that your eyes become more sensitive to light at night while you're driving. Some things are harder to prepare for, but when they, occur, they are easy to fix.

The same thing goes for your hearing. As you get older many people develop hearing loss. Some may have problems hearing high frequencies. While others may have difficulty understanding a normal speaking voice, you learn what precautions you can take to avoid most of this late-life hearing loss.

YOUR TEETH AND GUMS

Not everyone brushes their teeth every day which results in early tooth decay and the possibility of gingivitis and infection.

Typically, when you get older, you tend to develop dry mouth which can also lead to other dental problems.

YOUR SKIN

Do you see more wrinkles in your face? That's because of your skin changes as you age. A lot is going on with your skin, and we're going to discuss it in detail.

YOUR WEIGHT

Your weight can be a significant factor in how fast you age. As you get older, your metabolism slows down, and your body burns fewer calories. Almost everyone gains weight as they get older because they are not burning the calories due to decreased activity. We'll show you how to fix that problem.

LIFE EXPECTANCY

Remember in the beginning we talked about average life expectancy in the early 1900s was only 50 years old. As of 2018, the life expectancy on average in the United States is 80.1 years. It's 77.8 years for males and 82.3 years for females. Remember I said the average. That means that some must expire before the average age and others live longer than the average age. There are many contributing factors to why people die before reaching the average age. And will be discussing them later; however, what causes people to live longer than the average age is what you want to know.

Did you know that out of 224 countries, we are number 43 on the list for the longest longevity? That means that the average lifespan in 42 of the countries is longer than in the United States. The country of Monaco has the longest life expectancy which is 89 .4 years. That's 9.3 years longer than in the United States. The first question you ask is, what do they do differently in that country that allows them to live longer on average. We'll dissect that little later as well.

CAUSE AND EFFECT

Everything in life that we do has a cause and effect.

 If we eat and don't exercise, we get fat.

If we don't brush our, teeth, we get cavities and gingivitis.

If we eat the wrong, foods, we'll have other health issues.

If you want to live longer, you are going to have to change a few things. Not everyone's body is built the same; therefore, a person needs to customize their plan for longevity.

DON'T WAIT UNTIL YOU GET OLD

You can't wait until your body is already worn out; you have to start as early as you can.

You're going to have to set goals and meet them if you want to prolong your life beyond the average life expectancy.

LIVE TO BE 100

What do YOU have to do to live beyond a hundred years old?

There is no reason whatsoever you cannot prolong your life by following these simple steps So let' start with your:

MENTAL STATE:

From early childhood, you have been unconsciously exercising your brain. Early on while you were going to school you in a learning mode. You continue that mode until you got your first job. And then you went into a different kind of learning mode. Learning the job then you went into the reinforcement of keeping your brain sharp by performing the duties in your career. But then you retired. The first thing you wanted to do was forget everything you knew about the job you retired from. It's only the natural thing to do. But if you don't keep exercising your brain, your brain will begin to change. You can prolong the aging effect on your brain by keeping your mind active by:

1. Reading books and working crossword puzzles
2. Exercising. Exercising increases the blood flow to your brain. You should exercise a minimum of 30 minutes per day. You can walk, jog, bike, and do calisthenics
3. Eat brain food. Make sure your diet consists of foods that are healthy for your brain, Foods with high levels of omega-3. Fish oils from salmon mackerel tuna herring and sardines. Eat other foods like Dark chocolate which contains cocoa which is a flavonoid that makes it one type of an antioxidant. You can eat berries nuts and seeds. Eating whole grains is a good source of vitamin E. Caffeine helps keep you from feeling sleepy, and it also helps your brain process information. Drinking coffee is a good source of Antioxidants. Eggs are excellent brain food. They are a good source of vitamin B-6 and vitamin B-12. Vegetables that contain glycosylates which are Antioxidants. They include brussels sprouts cabbage cauliflower turnips and kale. In a

nutshell, Brain-boosting foods need to contain one or more of the following:

a. Antioxidants, such as flavonoids or vitamin E
b. B vitamins
c. Helpful fats
d. Omega fatty acids

In addition to having a healthy brain is essential to continually keep their mind active. If you think you're old, you will be old people who think they are younger than their actual age has a propensity to live longer.

DIET AND NUTRITION

Research has proven that a proper healthy diet solves most of the aging problems. By eating the right foods, in the right amounts is tremendously beneficial to all of your bodily functions.

Essential Vitamins and Minerals for People who are over 50 Include

Vitamin D

If you are age 51–70, you need at least 15 mcg (600 IU) each day, but not more than 100 mcg (4,000 IU).

If you are over age 70, you need at least 20 mcg (800 IU), but not more than 100 mcg (4,000 IU).

vitamin D comes from fatty fish, fish liver oils, fortified milk and milk products, and fortified cereals.

Vitamin B12

You need 2.4 mcg every day. Get it from meat, fish, poultry, milk, and fortified breakfast cereals. They may need to take vitamin B12 supplements and eat foods fortified with this vitamin.

Calcium

Men age 51-70 need 1,000 mg each day.

Men age 71 and older and women age 51 and older need 1,200 mg each day.

You shouldn't consume more than 2,000 mg each day. Calcium is essential for healthy bones and teeth. You can get calcium from milk, and other dairy foods, dark-green leafy vegetables, soybeans, sardines, and salmon may also contain calcium

Magnesium

Women age 51 and over need 320 mg each day. Men need 420 mg. You can find this mineral in foods containing dietary fiber, green leafy vegetables, whole grains, and nuts and seeds.

Potassium

For people age 51 and over, 4,700 mg per day is adequate. Foods high in potassium include dried apricots, lentils, and potatoes. milk, coffee, and tea may also contain potassium

Adults get a lot of their potassium from milk, coffee, tea, and other nonalcoholic beverages.

PHYSICAL FITNESS

Very few people who don't engage in physical activity live past their mid-60s. That's because of the living habits started from their mid-40s. Here's where it all begins. Your body should still be in good physical shape in your mid-40s and started in her early 50s your body begins to start the aging process. First your eyesight, and you need glasses. Now you're starting to think that you are beginning to get old, which you are. From this point on, you should never let that thought crossed your mind again. Remember, people who think they are younger than they actually are, tend to live longer. It's the power of positive thinking. You have to understand, what your body needs to do to keep the aging process at bay as long as possible. Remember these things.

1. Exercising helps the blood flow through your cardiovascular system. Which helps your heart and brain functions.
2. Exercising helps your digestive system functioning properly
3. Exercising burns calories and keeps your metabolism healthy
4. Exercising enables you to keep your muscles firm and elastic.

MAINTAIN A HEALTHY WEIGHT

One of the most important aspects of staying healthy is keeping your body at its proper weight. Use the chart below to determine your appropriate weight. And set your goal to gain that weight and maintain it.

Height	Weight		
	Normal	**Overweight**	**Obese**
4' 10"	91 to 118 lbs.	119 to 142 lbs.	143 to 186 lbs.
4' 11"	94 to 123 lbs.	124 to 147 lbs.	148 to 193 lbs.
5'	97 to 127 lbs.	128 to 152 lbs.	153 to 199 lbs.
5' 1"	100 to 131 lbs.	132 to 157 lbs.	158 to 206 lbs.
5' 2"	104 to 135 lbs.	136 to 163 lbs.	164 to 213 lbs.
5' 3"	107 to 140 lbs.	141 to 168 lbs.	169 to 220 lbs.
5' 4"	110 to 144 lbs.	145 to 173 lbs.	174 to 227 lbs.
5' 5"	114 to 149 lbs.	150 to 179 lbs.	180 to 234 lbs.
5' 6"	118 to 154 lbs.	155 to 185 lbs.	186 to 241 lbs.
5' 7"	121 to 158 lbs.	159 to 190 lbs.	191 to 249 lbs.
5' 8"	125 to 163 lbs.	164 to 196 lbs.	197 to 256 lbs.
5' 9"	128 to 168 lbs.	169 to 202 lbs.	203 to 263 lbs.
5' 10"	132 to 173 lbs.	174 to 208 lbs.	209 to 271 lbs.
5' 11"	136 to 178 lbs.	179 to 214 lbs.	215 to 279 lbs.
6'	140 to 183 lbs.	184 to 220 lbs.	221 to 287 lbs.
6' 1"	144 to 188 lbs.	189 to 226 lbs.	227 to 295 lbs.
6' 2"	148 to 193 lbs.	194 to 232 lbs.	233 to 303 lbs.

6' 3"	152 to 199 lbs.	200 to 239 lbs.	240 to 311 lbs.
6' 4"	156 to 204 lbs.	205 to 245 lbs.	246 to 320 lbs.
BMI	19 to 24	25 to 29	30 to 39

Source: National Institutes of Health. Don't see your weight? Learn more.

Obesity is the number one life-shortening disease in the world today. It is the root cause of most significant disabilities. Starting with your heart. Remember your heart has to circulate blood throughout your cardiovascular system, the more overweight your body is, the harder it is for your heart to pump blood to your system. Being overweight can cause most of the problems listed below

Heart disease and stroke, High blood pressure, High cholesterol, Diabetes, Osteoarthritis, Cancer., Gallbladder disease, and gallstones. Gout. Among other conditions

Additionally, obesity can cause breathing problems, such as sleep apnea (when a person stops breathing during sleep) and then maybe even asthma.

Many people who lived to be over a hundred years old have lived healthy lives, doing normal things. Nothing stands out that could cause them to live longer than anyone else. Some have smoked for their whole lives or chewed tobacco. Some drink alcohol every day. By the way, alcohol in moderation is supposed to be good for you. However, most of these individuals are exceptions. When researchers go out to locations where the population is known to live longer, they get a better look at the reasons why.

In Asian countries, like Japan that has a lot of centurions, the researchers find several things that might explain longevity.

1. The average diet is simple. And consist of fish, which is high in omega-3. Rice and vegetables. Most Asians are well within the weight limit for their height. And, finally, the meals they eat are balanced and nutritious because most of their food is steamed keeping in the nutrients. Very rarely do you see an overweight Asian.
2. Physical fitness. Most Asians live very active lives and either walked to where they're going or ride bicycles. It is not uncommon to see a 90-year-old woman or a man riding a bike.

But it would be scarce to see a person that old riding a bike in the United States.

THE SECRET TO LONGEVITY

IS NO SECRET AT ALL,

IT'S JUST COMMON SENSE

So, the answer to longevity is not so hard to understand. What is hard is changing your lifestyle if your goal is to live to be 100 years old. So here it is, below is exactly what you need to do to live to be 100 years old, assuming, of course, you're in good shape to start with.

1. **Brain** Keep your mind active, think positive thoughts
2. **Nutrition** Eat nutritious food in the proper portions
3. **Weight** Maintain your body weight based on your height
4. **Physical Fitness** Exercise your whole body regularly

MY ADVICE IS SIMPLE

My advice to you is simple if your middle age now. Then you have a shot at making it to 100. We only talked about the natural way of reaching a hundred. But with the medical advances that are occurring daily. Your chances of living to be over 100 are getting better every day. Modern medicine has produced wondrous drugs that do remarkable things to our body. Many of these drugs are preventative drugs that keep your body from deteriorating quicker than usual. Without these drugs, the life expectancy of many people in the United States would have been much less than what it is now.

The critical point here is, if you change your lifestyle now while you're in middle age, you may not need to use these drugs when you get older.

If you wish to further research the subject, further, I provided some links to websites that talk about your health and longevity and also a couple of YouTube videos that might be of interest. I

https://www.wikihow.com/Live-to-Be-100-Years-Old

https://www.rush.edu/health-wellness/quick-guides/what-is-a-healthy-weight

https://youtu.be/jIYPfjqwhFM

https://youtu.be/jIYPfjqwhFM

If you like what you read in this book and you think it might be of benefit to you, you might be interested in two of my other books. Here are the Amazon links.

KILLER PANIC ATTACKS

https://www.amazon.com/gp/product/B010WL454I/ref=dbs_a_def_rwt_bibl_vppi_i36

WHEN I KICK THE BUCKET: WHAT HAPPENS NEXT?

https://www.amazon.com/gp/product/B01
DMSUZ92/ref=dbs_a_def_rwt_bibl_vppi
_i46

I've written over 50 books, they are all published on Amazon. Use the following link to see all of the titles in one place.

https://www.amazon.com/BOBBY-F.-BROOKS/e/B00R1T8CYO%3Fref=dbs_a_mng_rwt_scns_share

Thank you very much for reading my book. And I hope the best for you